SURVIVING ALZHEIMER'S

A Guide for Families

by Florian Raymond

ELDER BOOKS

THE CAREGIVERS SERIES

Forest Knolls • California

**Library of Congress
Cataloging in Publication Data**

Main entry under title:
Surviving Alzheimer's
Raymond, Florian.

1. Alzheimer's disease. 2. Home care
3. Activities. 4. Aged-Home care
5. Nursing home care.

ISBN 0-943873-00-2

Printed in the United States of America
Cover Design: Bill Roarty

TABLE OF CONTENTS

ॐ

ACKNOWLEDGEMENTS

To my mother
whose indomitable spirit,
unwavering optimism and concern
for others triumphed over
the adversities of aging.

And to these very
special friends for
their support, encouragement
and invaluable assistance:

C. William Kipp, Ph.D.
Director, Social Work
Mt. Sinai Medical Center
Miami Beach, Florida

Deborah Hurwitz, L.C. S. W.
Clinical Counselor
Wien Center, Mt. Sinai
Medical Center
Miami Beach, Florida.

i

ट॰

PREFACE

You, dear caregiver, are not alone.

Statistics at this time cite 4 million Americans
suffering from Alzheimer's disease, with the
frightening prediction of over 14 million by 2040.
And for almost every patient, there is a caregiver
waging a daily battle against the insidious,
unrelenting cruelty of the disease.

Research is working tirelessly to discover the
causes of Alzheimer's and to develop new
treatments and more effective medications.
Although some progress has been made,
there is still no cure. But just as other grimly
resistant diseases were finally conquered, we
can only hope for the day when a cure will be
found for Alzheimer's, and our faith and
prayers will be answered.

Please note:
The generic "she" is used to designate
both male and female.

एक

INTRODUCTION
A WORD TO THE WEARY

Caregiving should be classified as a
noble profession. Unfortunately it has received
no status, no recognition. It is a labor of love
that usually falls to a female member of the
family, since women have always been the
primal nurturers. We are mothers, wives, sisters,
daughters...a legion of desperate women
struggling with the unknown. Many men are also
thrust into the caregiving role as they try gallantly
to cope with their spouses' illness.

From my personal experience and the input of
others in a similar situation, I know how
frightening, how despairing it is to watch the
gradual disintegration of a loved one. As the
disease progresses, the patient becomes more
dependent, more disoriented, more incapable
of self-care. Along with the physical, mental and
emotional impairments is the catastrophic loss

of self: someone who was and no longer is. Although at present there is no cure, there is hope and support at hand. There are coping skills to help you overcome your fears and lighten your burden – ways and means to make the going easier. For through it all, you are the only ray of light, the only semblance of reason and affirmation in your patient's fading existence. You make the quality of life more viable, more livable, more humane. Surely there is no greater love! And that's what survival is all about. ɜ❧

CARING FOR THE PATIENT

ॐ

ACTIVITIES FOR THE PATIENT

Activities help the person with Alzheimer's disease to succeed and enjoy moment-to-moment satisfaction. You can create many simple activities to relieve boredom and provide much needed stimulation. Chores and activities can be sensitively set at a level which does not place the person in a position of failure.

This chapter presents activity ideas which I have found useful. They can be used by the caregiver, the companion, the nurse's aide or the occasional visitor. Use your ingenuity to add to the list. By keeping the patient stimulated and involved, you can help slow the consequences of the disease.

Touch

Your relative needs to continue experiencing the warmth of person-to-person contact. Touch is perhaps the most eloquent communication tool we have and often speaks louder than words. A handclasp, a kiss, a hug — all tender benedictions to your patient and affectionate expressions of

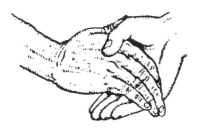

your love. Touch provides gentle healing that relieves tensions and anxieties. Use it often throughout the day to reassure your relative that you are there to comfort and care for her.

Massage

Use gentle massage to communicate love and caring. Get a basic guidebook from the library and teach yourself a simple technique. Start on the back, using circular motions. Move on to the arms and hands and end at the torso and feet. Remember that the patient's attention span is limited, so five or ten minutes at a time is sufficient.

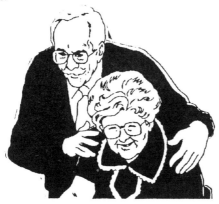

Music Makes The World Go Round

It's amazing what a familiar song can do, even for severely withdrawn patients. Feet start tapping, hands move—some begin to hum along and suddenly start singing the words, an astonishing feat! Music helps relieve tension for both patient and caregiver as this anecdote demonstrates:

Mrs Swanson: *Sometimes when we're riding in the car, my husband will insist upon repeating the same irritating conversation over and over until I'm ready to scream. But by turning up the volume on the radio I can 'tune out' the annoyance by listening to sweet, soothing music. That little ploy serves both of us very well.*

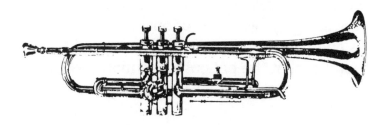

Music also activates memories of the distant past. Keep this in mind when you play those wonderful old favorites. Old time songs help stir recollections of the good times (and the sad ones) and in many cases elicit smiles and laughter. Music therapy is recognized as one of the potent treatments for depression, anxieties and many other mental and emotional illnesses. It is an ally in your battle to create a warmer, more loving environment for your relative.

The Caregivers Catalog, listed in Appendix 3, has several good music resources. **Big Band Gold** is a selection of recordings from superstars of the big band era and helps trigger memories of special moments and events. Listening to old hymns is often comforting and a musical selection such as **Hymns of Gold** (the Caregiver's Catalog) can help your relative while away the time peacefully.

The Children's Hour

Strange title? But just look at what's happened. Suddenly, you have become the parent, and your parent the child. This role reversal is the poignant effect of cognitive loss and progressive deterioration. The dependency of your loved one becomes a fearful responsibility. The one who once cuddled you, tended to your needs with loving heart and hands, who was always there to comfort you has gone back in time. The relationship has come full circle, dear caregiver, and it's your turn now.

Down Memory Lane

The past is more familiar to the person with Alzheimer's disease than the present. Strangely, the happenings of long ago transcend the reality of the here and now. So make the most of the past and use it to reminisce with your relative.

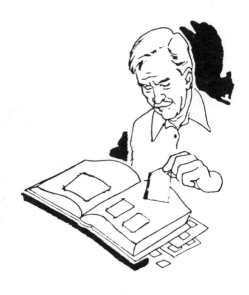

Take out the photo album and recall the events
that once made life so special, so endearing.
There's a well of loveliness stored in those
precious memories from the past. You could be
well rewarded with your loved one's happy reaction
and also enjoy a good time yourself. Many patients
enjoy watching old time movies which you can rent
at your local video store. Listening to old time
radio programs is also popular and these are aired
periodically. Two audio kits which I have found
useful are **Radio's Greatest Moments** and **Radios
Greatest Comedies.** These are tapes of radio's
finest moments in drama, newscasts, golden
comedy and the great radio commercials.
Available through the Caregiver's Catalog, these
tapes make a treasure house of enjoyable
memories.

What A Difference A Day Makes

Especially at the Day Care Center. With attentive supervision, patients participate in various planned activities designed to stimulate and energize. It's amazing to see a lethargic, withdrawn patient suddenly join in a sing-along, or get up to dance with a partner. The Center provides a congenial, caring environment that stimulates interaction and encourages mobility and expression with carefully selected exercises and games. Lunch and snacks are served, and the day's program of education, recreation and entertainment keeps patients pleasantly occupied. A very productive experience for the patient; a tremendous relief for the caregiver.

A Pet By Any Other Name

It could be a dog, a cat, or even a pet bird. Pets fulfill the human desire to be needed and satiate the deep-seated hunger for affection and tactile communication.

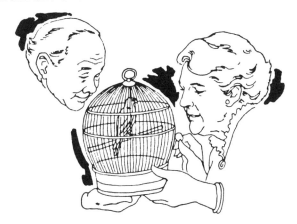

By providing a pet, you fill a void in a life that is suffering cognitive loss and other afflictions. At the same time, you are giving your loved one a sense of peace and happiness of immense therapeutic value. Since there are no rules for taking care of and helping Alzheimer's patients with their disabilities, you must trust your own judgement. I believe there is only one golden rule: if it works, use it ...with blessing!

Doll Therapy

"Doll therapy" became a small miracle for me in caring for my mother and to my knowledge I was the first one to advocate it. Since pets were being used to ease the tensions and restrictions of Alzheimer's, I reasoned a doll would achieve the same results, when using a pet was not feasible.

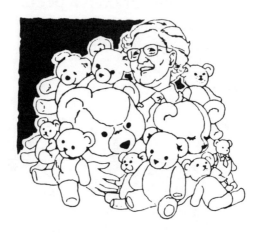

My mother always had a special fondness for dolls, so I bought her the kind she could relate to:

a blue-eyed baby girl with lovely blond curls and a delicately molded face. (Mother was not of the cabbage patch era!). The doll seemed to answer an unspoken, but deeply human desire to be needed, and mother responded with loving care. She called the doll "Julie" (although I never discovered where that name came from.) Now Julie became one of the family. Mother would talk to her, cuddle her, go to sleep with her nestled protectively in her arms. She even changed the doll's clothes from the little wardrobe I assembled. All of this contributed to mother's mobility and provided an absorbing, enjoyable activity that was stimulating. It was an intimate relationship that effected its gentle magic and frankly brought tears to my eyes.

I've watched impaired women who rarely uttered a word talk to a doll and cuddle it as though it were a live baby. Perhaps it evoked dormant memories of caring for a child from some distant long-ago in the dim recesses of their minds.

My credo for caregivers is: if it works, use it! — and don't worry about how unusual or unorthodox the idea is. There are no givens regarding definitive treatments of Alzheimer's patients; using creative ingenuity is sometimes all we have. And these simple activities can make a big difference! As for doll therapy, I have since learned that it is being used in nursing homes and other facilities for selected patients.

Back to Basics

Patients benefit from a daily schedule of physical exercises. Even sedentary patients can exercise in a chair by moving feet back and forth, stretching arms, kneading a soft rubber ball between the hands. These motions stimulate circulation and help people to function independently.

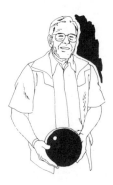

At first, there may be resistance, but persistence (or should I say infinite patience?) usually wins out. The effort is well worth it, especially for the patient's health.

Reading

Reading, a shared activity, provides moments of pleasant relaxation. Lately, there has been increased interest in stories and books which are particularly suited to people with memory problems. These stories feature uncomplicated themes and easily identifiable characters. Patients have been observed listening intently to the reader, obviously absorbed and alert.

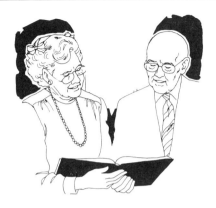

This must surely help to broaden the short attention span and engage interest in a stimulating way. For both of you this activity provides calm and comfort.

Declaration Of Independence

It's vitally important that you allow the patient to perform any activity she can still do for herself. It will elevate her self-esteem and create a feeling of productivity. Many very well-intentioned caregivers take over to the point where the patient expects constant attention. This is a disservice to both of you. What's more, it destroys your loved one's initiative and encourages more dependency.

Sure there are problems. As one caregiver complained: "If I let my sister dress herself she'll put her clothes on over her nightgown, and her shoes on the wrong feet." Certainly it's tiring and upsetting to have to redress her. But by nurturing your relative's independence, you are in fact helping her to remain active and in control for a longer period of time. 🙋

ᔚ

COPING WITH
DIFFICULT BEHAVIORS

Alzheimer's disease presents many difficult behavior patterns. Just as no two fingerprints are the same, each person presents different problems. What works for one might not be effective for another. Unfortunately there is no cure now, and only very generalized guidelines. So the caregiver must learn to trust her own observations and insight concerning the patient's care.

As the disease progresses, the patient's behavior patterns may range from the bizarre to the unacceptable. You must be aware of fluctuations in behavior and develop strategies to prevent everyday situations from developing into crises. This section describes how caregivers learned to handle difficult situations with creative applications of ingenuity. With plain common sense and a blessed sense of humor, you too will learn to respond to negative behavior with positive action. Some problems can be solved quickly; others call for infinite patience and understanding.

Agitation

The patient may become worried and agitated for no apparent reason, exhibiting bewildering mood swings and anxieties. This is often the direct effect of rapidly occurring physiological changes. Mental and physical abilities may deteriorate as the patient becomes increasingly dysfunctional.

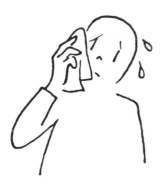

Sandra Smith: *I used to take my mother to the beauty parlor to have her hair done. But the past few times were a disaster. She kept complaining about everything: the water was too cold, the rollers too tight; the dryer too hot. All in a loud angry voice that was obviously disturbing to the other patrons. I understood when the manager politely asked me to please not bring her anymore, even though she apologized profusely and expressed how sorry she was for both of us. Now I do mother's hair myself. There are very few complaints and of course, no one else around to bother. So it's much easier for me, too.*

What You Can Do

- Acknowledge the expressed anxiety without referring to its source. Be calm and reassuring.

- Distract the patient by changing the subject or focusing her attention on something else.

- Anti-anxiety and other medications are available to help a severely distressed patient. Have your physician prescribe the appropriate medication.

Wandering

Wandering, particularly in the evening, is a common problem. Known as Sundowner's Syndrome, those affected become unusually energetic and disturbed about eight or nine in the evening. The danger of injury and of becoming lost is so great that every precaution must be taken to avoid the problem before it arises.

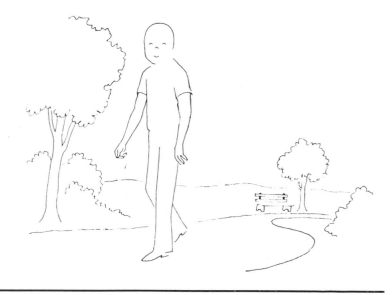

Susan Orthello: *I went into the kitchen for a few minutes to get some juice for my father. When I got back to the living room, he was gone. I was frantic. It was ten o'clock at night and I was all alone. I called the police and within an hour they brought him back. They found him walking (in his pajamas) down a dark side street near our home. They advised me to get a bracelet listing his name, address, and phone number. I took care of it the next day, and considered myself very lucky that no harm had come to him.*

There is no known cause for Sundowner's Syndrome, but the following guidelines can help you deal with this affliction.

What You Can Do

- Involve the patient in a regular daily program of recreational and physical activities to help him sleep better at night.

- Create a special 'wandering' area within your home where the patient is free to pace as he wants.

- If wandering becomes a serious problem, have electronic devices installed which will alert you when the person is leaving the house.

- Contact your local Alzheimer's Association and obtain an I.D bracelet.

- Have a clear, recent photo of your relative available at all times.

Inappropriate Sexual Behavior

Changes in sexuality often accompany Alzheimer's disease. For some, the sex drive is lessened. Other patients experience a renewed interest in sex. Occasionally, inappropriate sexual behavior occurs such as masturbating in public or making sexual advances to strangers, but this is not very common. When it happens, it causes much pain and embarrassment for family members, as this story illustrates:

Mrs. Brown: *We've had the same cleaning woman for many years, so I thought it strange when she told me she wouldn't be coming back anymore. "Why?" I asked mystified. She flushed and then stammered, "When you went to the store your father grabbed me and wanted me to go to bed with him." I felt terrible and tried to explain that he really didn't mean it; that he was sick and not himself. But she refused to listen and left. The next day a friend came to visit. When I went into the kitchen for coffee, she told me later that my father had made advances to her. Being an intelligent, informed woman, she handled it very well by ignoring his conduct and directing his attention to the TV. I guess someone else would call my poor father a 'dirty old man', but I know his preoccupation with sex is a sad manifestation of his illness and I'm heartsick about it. I spoke to his doctor who prescribed a medication that is supposed to relieve the problem.*

What You Can Do

- Use touch frequently in your everyday interactions with the patient. What the patient craves is not always sexual contact, but warm compassionate touch.

- If the patient undresses in public, check his clothing for comfort. Sometimes this behavior simply indicates discomfort.

- If sexual behavior suddenly becomes very inappropriate, check the patient's medication. If it has recently been changed, contact your physician and have the dose reduced or the medication changed entirely.

Doubting The Facts

Sometimes the Alzheimer's patient is quick to doubt the facts and any attempt at logical explanation is vehemently resisted. Reason plays no part in this no-win predicament— which makes it exceedingly difficult for caregivers.

John Scally: *Staring at the woman in the picture, my wife asked: "Who is she?" Lisa, our daughter, I answered. "You're lying," she shouted, "that's your girlfriend!" Rather than try to reason with her (it wouldn't matter anyway), I took the picture away and handed her a book on gardening, something she used to enjoy. She sat down and looked through the book as though nothing had taken place. The technique of focusing her attention on something else works like a charm.*

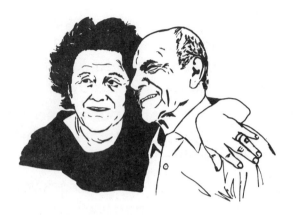

What You Can Do

- Change the subject immediately and involve the patient in an activity that requires a little physical effort, like walking into the kitchen for a snack or turning on some music to dissipate the tension.

- Discuss a special occasion that the patient participated in a long time ago. The past is sometimes amazingly clear to the patient, unlike the hazy present.

Forgetfulness

Memory deterioration usually occurs early in the disease. A patient who has just finished dinner will complain: "I haven't eaten all day!" Phone calls and visits from friends and relatives will not be remembered, with the patient saying bitterly, "No one ever comes here." Forgetfulness touches almost every phase of daily life, with family members enduring various angry charges of neglect: "You don't care about me!" Any loss is sad and unfortunate, but loss of memory is one of the hardest to bear... especially when retrogression takes place and the patient no longer recognizes her loved ones.

Jill Reider: *My mother accuses me of never visiting her, even though I see her every day. I've tried to explain, but to no avail. She has round-the-clock aides who try to console me with the explanation that she is very disoriented and is not responsible for what she says or does. I've cried about that and tried to resign myself to the situation, realizing that my mother is no longer aware of reality. I feel that I've lost my mother, that the mother I loved and knew is gone and I grieve as though she were dead.*

What You Can Do

- Use photographs to remind the patient of the important people in her life. Named photos of regular visitors help her stay in touch.

- Accept that although the patient's memory is impaired, there are still many loving ways you can reach her. Using touch, music and reminiscence are just some examples.

- Support whatever cognitive functions remain through a simple technique called reality orientation. This involves reminding the patient in an un-intrusive way of her own identity and of people and events in her life.

Suspicion

Insecurities and infirmities beset the patient to the point where almost everything is perceived as threatening and hostile. Angry accusations are often directed to the caregiver or anyone viewed as suspect: "You took my money"..."You stole my ring"... "What did you do with my coat?" The "accused" must try to deal with this volatile situation with a calm, assured confidence, never allowing the barrage of blame to shake her patience or her resolve to quietly clear the air. It becomes a test of endurance for the caregiver to maintain her equilibrium through every problem. But it becomes easier when you understand that these outbursts are involuntary; consequences of an illness that is merciless, to both patient and caregiver.

Mrs. Monroe: *My mother is suspicious of everyone, including me. Today she demanded I 'return the money' she said was missing from her purse. Trying to reason with her was a total failure, so I just changed the subject and started talking to her about events that were deeply rooted in her past. She responded so well that it was positively eerie. Of course, the 'missing money' was temporarily forgotten. I know it's the illness speaking, not my mother, but the cold evidence of her deterioration makes me depressed.*

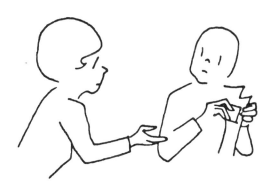

What You Can Do

- Introduce another topic that she can relate to: a forthcoming visit from a grandchild or a favorite relative.

- Give her a reassuring hug letting her know that you love her and that "everything is all right."

- If there is an item in the paper that might interest her, read it!

Embarrassing Social Behavior

Odd behaviors create off-the-wall situations that are difficult to control and socially unacceptable. Since they can't be foreseen, the caregiver must handle these sudden eruptions as best she can. Usually outings become less frequent as the caregiver anticipates the worst.

Rita Stokes: *I took my mother to the movies thinking she'd enjoy the change. She sat quietly for a while, then began to fidget and squirm in her seat. Suddenly she shouted at the screen, "Oh there's Lenny. Lenny. Lenny, come here!" I could sense everyone staring at us, my face hot with embarrassment. "Please watch the picture, Mother," I whispered. "I don't like it!" she shouted. I tried to leave with her but discovered she'd dropped her glasses and kicked off one shoe. After we found her things, we hastily left. I don't know what triggered her outburst, and I still don't know who 'Lenny' is, unless he reminded her of someone way back when. Alzheimer's plays strange tricks on all of us.*

What You Can Do

- If appropriate, quietly but firmly take the patient away from the scene. Don't be too upset; most people understand a problem that is obviously an unfortunate condition.

- Just because the episode occurred doesn't mean it will happen every time. You might try again, with positive results.

Aggression

A patient who rails at a locked door may become exceedingly overwrought, almost violent. In her distorted mind, the door becomes a barrier that threatens her freedom and locks her inside. Simply handing her the key can allay those fears. By unlocking the door the patient also senses she is free to leave. Usually at this point the patient doesn't exhibit any further desire to go outside.

Joan Woods: *Last night my husband ran to the front door and began banging on it, shouting furiously, "Let me out! Let me out." I was terribly upset but knew I must distract him. As calmly as possible, I approached him with the key in my hand. "We'll go out together," I said, opening the door. He looked at me for a moment, then turned away and went back into the living room. I believe that when he saw he could go out he no longer felt locked in. I breathed a sigh of relief as another crisis was managed – for now, anyway.*

What You Can Do

- Consult the doctor immediately where aggressive behavior is involved. Sometimes new medication may be responsible for drastic mood fluctuations.

- If the medication must be changed again, the patient may have to be hospitalized to observe her reactions.

- If the problem persists and you cannot deal with it, consider a day care program or nursing home for the patient. ‰

୬

CHILDREN AND ALZHEIMER'S

What Do You Tell Them

Gran has always been Amy's special friend. The one who cuddled her, read to her, tied her hair ribbons and brought her pretty gifts. But now Gran is not the same one Amy knew. This Gran looks at her in a funny way, and keeps asking the same question over and over. Puzzled, little six-year-old Amy answers, "I already told you that, Gran" and Gran shouts angrily, "Bad girl. Bad Girl!" Amy dissolves into tears while her mother tries to comfort her. "Gran isn't feeling well today, darling. She doesn't mean that. You know she loves you." But Amy refuses to be pacified. "I like my other Gran better," she sobs, burying her face in her mother's dress.

Unfortunately, situations like this can't be avoided, but they mustn't rupture already strained family relationships. As long as possible, try to keep visits active. Days will vary, circumstances change, but grandchildren have been the focal point of a grandparent's life. And somewhere within the shattered psyche are remnants of a love that can't be expressed or demonstrated. But they are there, just another casualty of the affliction. Surprisingly, a child can learn to accept the altered persona with reassurances that although there are bad days, there are good days too. And love for Gran makes all of them better.

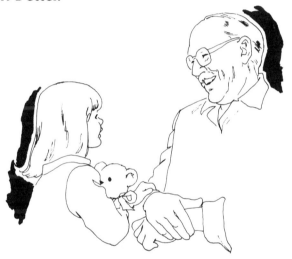

Help children understand the disease. There are many helpful books on the market which explain the disease process to children in an un-threatening way. **"Grandpa Doesn't Know It's Me"** has been found helpful by many families. Another book which has been highly acclaimed is **"Sachismo Means Happiness"**. Both books are available from the address listed in Appendix 2. ❧

ôù

MAKING LIFE EASIER

This chapter describes tips and techniques for making your job as caregiver easier. These guidelines are a result of my own personal experience as a caregiver. Although they have worked for me, they may not be useful with all patients. Just as no two fingerprints are the same, each patient presents different problems— what works for one might not be effective for another. Unfortunately, there is no cure now, and only very generalized guidelines. So you must learn to trust your own observations and insight concerning the care of your relative.

Doubt and Denial

Perhaps you are still caught in the cycle of doubt and denial. You manage to downplay odd behaviors and actions, and convince yourself there's nothing wrong. This is natural — we all seek refuge in denial for a time: "Mother's getting older, that's all. Older people are restless and become forgetful." But the strange actions persist:

your mother insists that she hasn't eaten all day when in fact she's just finished dinner. She berates you for taking her jewelry and accuses the delivery boy of stealing her groceries. Occasional hallucinatory episodes occur: she insists there's a strange man on the porch when it's clear there's no one there. At this stage, you can no longer refuse to recognize the emergency. Your mother is ill and needs a complete physical and mental examination to ascertain her condition.

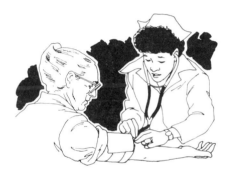

Only then can a therapeutic program be designed to help her and you through the trials ahead. At this point your relationship changes from mother and daughter to patient and caregiver. And so it came to all of us.

This Too Shall Pass

Crises are an unavoidable part of caregiving life. Our vulnerability and frustration seem to magnify every complication to disaster-status. When a change in medication produces adverse side effects, we panic, perceiving it as our personal failure. And nothing could be further from the truth. With each upset, I went through a cycle of guilt and recrimination. Self-reproach and recriminations have no place in this scenario. As time went on, my mother's illness taught me resilience and the importance of maintaining a balanced mental attitude: to accept each challenge with the saving grace and knowledge of that wonderful saying, "this too shall pass."

The Guilt Trap

Ambivalent feelings occur to everyone caring for an emotionally and physically unstable patient. As you face problems which have no immediate answers, your spirit is tested repeatedly. There is a very thin line between love and hate when difficult circumstances give rise to churning emotions. As the burden of caregiving escalates, resentment grows. Then you suffer the torment of secret shame for allowing such disloyal feelings to surface.

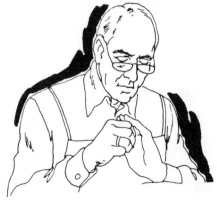

Remember that you've got enough on your shoulders without adding the burden of guilt. When you feel overwhelmed and resentful, it is because you are a stressed-out human being, subject to the frailties and weaknesses that beset all of us living under overwhelming pressures. This is a time to be gentle with yourself and find loving ways to replenish.

The Safety Zone

Statistics prove that most accidents happen in the home. To make your home as accident-proof as possible:

- Take up all area rugs that are skid-prone;
- Remove all objects that could be easily displaced and fall;
- Install grab bars in bathrooms and other areas to avoid tripping;
- Keep scissors, knives and other sharp instruments hidden;
- Leave floors unwaxed to provide safer footing.

Those are just a sample of the more obvious hazards, but there are many more that demand safety precautions to avoid serious accidents. As for your safety zone, it could be your room or any private little area where you can retreat for some quiet rest and relaxation. "Safe and sane" seems to acquire a meaningful interpretation here.

Enjoying Love and Laughter

There's too little of it in our lives. But when an occasional incident produces its own humorous result, that's cause for celebration and a welcome moment of shared laughter and pleasure. This caregiver recalls a humorous event with obvious delight:

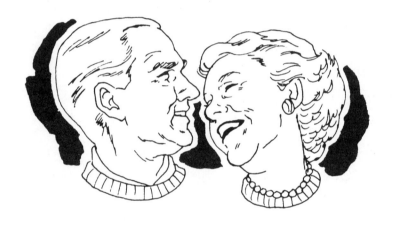

Shirley Day: *My mother called me into the bedroom in real panic. "Look at how much weight I've gained," she wailed. I looked... and burst into laughter. My mother, who wears a full size 16 had somehow managed to squeeze herself into my size 6 nightgown. When I explained why the gown didn't fit, she laughed heartily, greatly relieved. It was worth the rare carefree moment we enjoyed together!*

Small Changes

Small changes are sometimes welcome. You might discover that certain changes in the routine can make a difference: like serving a meal on a tray table in the living room to whet a waning appetite; or taking "wheel chair walks" outdoors for a very welcome change of scene.

Although routine is all-important for the person with Alzheimer's, it is also true that 'variety is the spice of life.' A fresh locale (even though it's in the home) can make a routine procedure more interesting. Introducing something new — perhaps a small bouquet on the table or a colorful new robe — can effect a kind of response-stimulation.

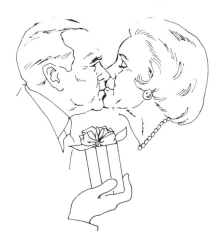

Anything that will activate the patient is worth a try. Use your common sense to decide when changes in the routine are appropriate. All you can do is make your patient's life more livable with your diligence and concern. No one could do more!

Knowing When To Let Well-Enough Alone

Too often, as over-solicitous caregivers, we keep on doing what is "right" or "expected" for our patients when letting well enough alone would be preferable. Learning to distinguish the difference and act accordingly makes it easier for both patient and caregiver.

Geraldine Ryan: *My sister went to bed fully clothed, right down to her shoes. There was a time b.c. (before caregivers) when I wouldn't let that go by: I would have awakened her to undress and get into nightclothes. But now I looked at her sleeping peacefully and tiptoed out of the room. My decision was the result of intelligent awareness-guidance from my support counselor. My sister and I are both benefitting from my learning experience.*

Being Adaptable

As a hands-on caregiver, I learned to adapt, to innovate and to use plain common sense when nothing else seemed to make sense. Problems kept cropping up. Like the shower problem that emerged one morning. My mother suddenly seemed upset as though the routine had become an assault, even though she'd always enjoyed it. Then it occurred to me that standing under the spray (which was hard to adjust) required too much effort for her. This time, the remedy was simple. A shower chair and hand-held portable that permitted control of the flow kept mother comfortable and made bathing easier. The message is simple: when the old way of doing things no longer works, try a new way!

White Lies

A friend was expressing her regret at having to lie to her husband. "He kept asking when our son would visit". "Finally I told him that Mike would be here in the afternoon, even though he was really out of town. I've never lied to my husband before and it bothers me, even though he'll forget it, for awhile, anyway."

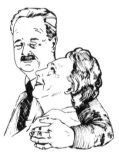

Sometimes the only way to deal with the patient's anxiety is to tell a white lie. It can be a survival strategy. My friend's response appeased her husband and gave her some relief at the same time.

Whatever the strategy, use it! You are laboring with very abnormal behaviors that require unusual handling. You are to be complimented for your insight and sensitivity. Soothing your relative's anxieties is mutually beneficial and layers a potentially irritating situation with calm reassurance.

Nothing Is Written In Stone

When you got up this morning, you knew you couldn't face all the procedures that had to be done, especially with your energy level at a new low. The solution: quietly determine only what is absolutely essential and adjust your schedule. Substitute a quick sponge for the time-consuming bath; serve cold cereal instead of hot; serve a fruit and sandwich lunch and forego some of the extras for a change. One day isn't going to make a big difference in your relative's life. Practically, it won't even be noticed. But it will make a big difference to you in terms of easing the workload and lifting morale. ❧

કર્

CARING FOR YOUR SELF

❧

Renewing Yourself

You will need regular time-out from the daily grind of caregiving to re-charge. Work out a schedule which will allow you time for outside diversions and stick to it. Otherwise, as a 24-hour caregiver, you will be in dire trouble right from the start. And certainly less able to manage your duties than one who plans activities, with the resultant benefits of warm relationships and interaction with family and friends. Enlist a relief helper: perhaps a family member, a friend or an aide. This will make life a little easier.

Self-preservation qualifies as your number one priority. Especially when your own life is almost inextricably meshed with your patient's existence. Eating on the run; cancelling doctor's appointments; forgetting to take your own medications and vitamins; all wreak havoc for the caregiver who neglects herself. Consider them danger signals with serious consequences. There are times when you must become your own priority and here are some ways and means to achieve it.

Only One Day At A Time

Familiar phrase. Just six well-chosen words that have helped millions get through the dark side of life. Acknowledging only one day at a time can **buy** time. Focusing the boundaries of your perception into this compact span gives you some breathing time: today is the day; tomorrow is far away, and yesterday is past. Perhaps you're still fretting over something that you feel should have been done, but was left unresolved. Just forget it! Past-tense worrying is an abysmal waste of time and energy, cluttering your mind with so much mental debris. Clean your mental house and get on with it. Small consolation is the fact that there will always be something to worry about, if you let it.

The Quick Fix

It's done with imagery, a wonderful source of do-it-yourself escapism. Imagine your favorite spot. Maybe it's a tranquil lake bordered with tall fragrant pines, crystal water rippling on a pebbled shore, a silver sun glinting through soft, cushiony clouds. Maybe it's a cherished event that evokes deep-down joy. There are treasured moments throughout life that will never be forgotten; memories that conjure up shining reminiscences of love and laughter. Bring 'em back alive, to be lived and loved all over again.

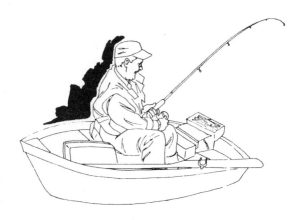

Laughter Lights Up Your Life

It's the best medicine! You've heard that, of course. Norman Cousins extolled the virtues of laughter in his book "Anatomy of An Illness," in which laughter played a major role in his recovery from a devastating illness.

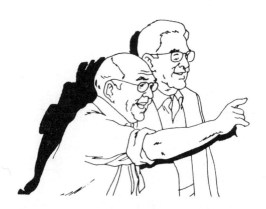

The benefits of laughter have been documented by the medical profession, and universally acclaimed as a contributory factor to healing. Studies reveal that laughter strengthens the immune system and helps to alleviate depression and defuse tensions. It's hard to laugh when you feel trapped within the confines of a tragic illness, but there are times when a good laugh can clear the air and restore harmony. A sense of humor is a blessed attribute. Apply generously and use often!

The Wizard of Nods

An occasional catnap during a trying day does wonders for revitalizing body and mind. Eleanor Roosevelt was one of our more famous catnapers, and there is a long list of prominent celebrities who attest to the instant pickup they enjoy with a short siesta. The trick is to relax your tense muscles and close your eyes.

The Mini Vacation

This category embraces a wide range of little diversions. Take a ride to visit someone you haven't seen lately; a trip to an art gallery, museum or new shopping mall. Browse through an interesting book store, or check out a new movie. Anything that will brighten and lighten your day can break the rigid monotony of routine.

The Walkie-Talkie

Combine the exhilarating effects of a brisk walk with the pleasure of a one-on-one communication with a friend. Fortunately, walking does not require special outfits, expensive equipment, or a specified place.

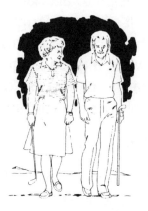

Take a walk around the park, the beach... through
a shopping mall, and talk to your heart's content.
It's really surprising how much enjoyment and
sheer physical and mental release can be obtained
from a few well-spent hours outdoors.

The Minor Miracle

Treat yourself to a new hairdo, get a manicure, a
pedicure...indulge in the heavenly toning of a
massage. It's amazing what only a few hours
dedicated solely to yourself can do for your
appearance, your psyche and your self-confidence.

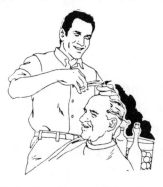

And you won't need a mirror to confirm the gratifying results. You'll know it's even better, you'll show it! Knowing that you look well will shore up your self-esteem and lift sagging spirits. You'll find caregiving easier with this enhanced attitude.
For the male caregiver, a visit to the barber, an afternoon of golf or cards will produce the same invigorating impact. In short, be good to yourself. You deserve it!

Music Hath Charms

It soothes, evokes delightful memories, and chases away the blues. Play your favorite tapes, kick off your shoes...just relax and listen.

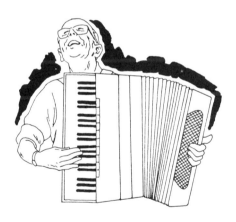

These special moments add up to instant refreshment. Music therapy has become a formidable influence in overcoming depressions, improving mental illness and other afflictions. Music is a universal language, talking in every tongue, understood by every listener.

Tea For Two

When it's impossible for you to get out, arrange a simple lunch for you and a friend. Enjoying each other's company with a heart-to-heart can be a poignant, emotional release and great picker-upper.

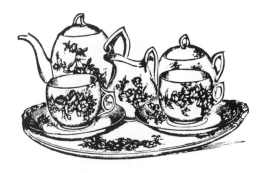

Keeping in touch with friends and outside interests is of the utmost importance. It will prevent you from becoming a shut-in, removed from relationships and contacts that are essential to overcoming the stresses of caregiving.

The Good Housekeeping Seal of Disapproval

You earn it when you're stuck in a rut with household duties. Let us count the ways: moaning over unmade beds ("they make me feel sloppy")...agonizing over unwaxed floors...worrying because the laundry wasn't done on Tuesday ("I always did it on Tuesday") etc. etc. This useless pursuit of trivia is of insignificance in relation to your first concern: your relative's well-being. And if a day dawns when the laundry can't be done and the windows are streaked and the floors scuffed...so what?

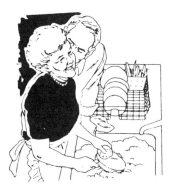

Just think of the Don Quixote syndrome and relax. Realize those windows are only in your mind. Then take a breath... a deep breath and loosen up. Recall the irrefutable retort of the maid who was scolded for not dusting the window sills: "This house gonna last longer than us." How true!

Have You Discovered Your Library Lately?

If not, now's a very good time. Read the best-sellers, delve into psychology, poetry, the arts, current events. It's all there on those richly laden shelves that include a dazzling variety of record albums, tapes and cassettes.

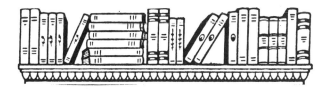

In the calm and peaceful atmosphere of the library you'll find yourself succumbing to the soothing effect of a tranquil environment. And since most libraries present interesting programs, movies, book reviews and lectures, you can keep up with the times with occasional refreshing visits. You need this special get-away to nourish your mind and to forget your cares.

The Wheel Of Misfortune

It grinds on relentlessly, with the exhausted caregiver rotating in a chaotic scramble of endless chores. Stop the world and get off! Take five.... luxuriate in a warm bath; do a few exercises; phone a friend. Your energy level will rise; your blood pressure will fall. That will take care of now.... this hectic moment. But now is only one day at a time. Live it that way: one day at a time, without looking back or looking ahead. Sometimes, anticipation can be worse than realization.

Beat The Burnout Blues

Occasional burnout happens to everyone. But more to the overstressed, over-extended caregiver, easy prey to illness. That's when taking care of yourself is a practical necessity. Realize that you need help and do something about it immediately. Engage a friend, relative, or an aide to make it possible for you to take a few hours away on a regular basis. There may come a time when illness will incapacitate you for awhile, and outside assistance will be absolutely needed. At first, your relative may not accept the arrangement willingly;

it may take several attempts before it becomes familiar and feasible, but be determined. You're saving another life....<u>yours.</u>

Tell It To Your Buddy

Yes, the buddy system is alive and well. When your world goes haywire and there's no relief in sight, turn to the telephone.

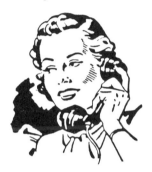

There's always a sympathetic, understanding person on the other end: a close friend, relative or member of your support group. Talk it out; you'll feel better as soon as you get back on track with the comfort of release. This is one of those instant therapies that should rate high priority on every caregiver's emergency list.

Bridge Over The River Cry

We've all cried a torrent on days when nothing seems to be working out. But with infusions of hope and courage we can bridge that seemingly insurmountable frustration and keep going. It's not easy; seems like we're constantly being tested for our patience and endurance.

However, crying is a safety valve, a natural mechanism that relieves the stifling pressures and suffocating build-up of clogged emotions. Yes, you can cry if you want to; it's your problem...and it'll help. A 'good cry' has therapeutic benefits; sometimes it's the only outlet we have. But keep in mind that tomorrow is another day, a brand new day and it could be much better. Keep the faith and hang in there!

Be Wise-Exercise

There's always walking — it's easily available to all of us. And then there are all the other options for improving circulation and providing refreshing activity: Yoga, aerobic videos, how-to books, stationary bikes...the list goes on and on. (Not to forget the virtues of plain old housework, duties which hardly qualify for the glamour-league of calisthenics, but are not a bad substitute in a pinch.)

Make exercise a part of your daily ritual. This attention to bending, stretching and deep, deep breathing will pay very attractive dividends and they're all yours!

Food For Thought

Food is one of the basic necessities of life. Yet how much time do we spend evaluating what is "good" for us, or more importantly, what we need in order to feel well. It can't be done alone. But there are highly qualified nutritionists who can prepare a complete workup and analysis of your body-condition. Using hair samples, blood tests and other diagnostic procedures, they assess what nutrients you are lacking; also what foods to avoid in order to obtain optimum health. Your health is what their profession is all about.

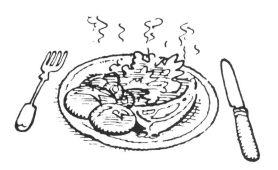

Proper nutrition and vitamin therapy have achieved dramatic improvement in mental, emotional and even physical disabilities for many. Both patient and caregiver could benefit greatly from customized diets specially designed to personal requirements. Surely anything as progressive and constructive is worth a try. You might discover dramatic results.

No Fuss, No Muss

Talk about short-cuts! Just a visit to your supermarket or favorite food store and you're home, free from cooking! All you do is select attractive, nutritious frozen food dinners that are available in every dietary requirement: salt-free, low-fat, cholesterol-free.

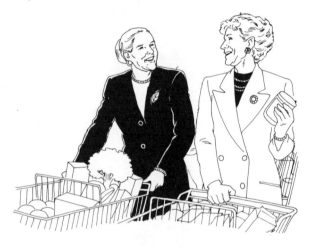

Best of all, it makes an occasional meal work-free with dishes that provide tasty menus, allowing you extra time when you need it most. Making life easier pays off in what I term the convenience-connection. Use it often.

Spirituality and Actuality

Some inner strength, fueled by profound belief transcends the harsh bitterness of reality into an uplifted state of higher consciousness. However it is attained, this transition gives the caregiver blessed respite from daily trials.

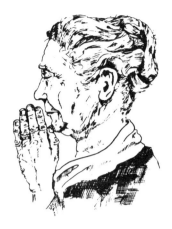

A religious service, meditating, or listening to tapes helps relieve tension and instills feelings of hope and encouragement. This affirmation of spiritual self-help overcomes despair and futility. When you discover what it is that produces this magical state of deliverance, it will become your own palliative, your personal good luck charm of faith and forbearance.

What Friends Are For

Don't try to be too independent, like a one-man band fighting a frightening battle all alone. Shutting yourself away will only make you feel more isolated and depressed. Becoming a martyr doesn't solve problems; it creates them. Allow a little leaning once in a while. Friends are one of life's real blessings. Those understanding people who gather round when the storm clouds break, who are there when you need a listening ear or a helping hand.

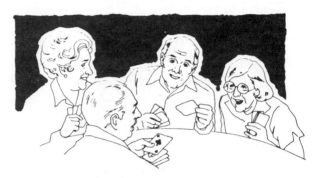

And who are always ready to pitch in, no matter what. Tell people practical ways in which they can help, such as giving you relief one night per month to go to a movie, coming over to visit, phoning your relative weekly. People often disappear out of awkwardness; they don't know how to handle the situation.

By giving friends guidelines for helping, you ensure that your relative and you will not be isolated.

Lighten Up!

Caregivers who give their all and become deadly serious with their responsibilities face health-threatening consequences. A sense of humor helps you weather the rough spots. While this in no way attempts to minimize the gravity of Alzheimer's, it is an honest effort to maximize your chances of survival as a whole person. Balance problems and pleasures so that the scale remains equally weighted in both directions. And if that sounds unattainable, just remember: a little pleasure goes a long way!

Enjoy The Moment

That very special moment, presaged by a surprise phone call, an unexpected letter, an exciting invitation. The kind of extraordinary happening that exhilarates and thrills the spirit. Savor the full flavor with total absorption, allowing nothing to mar its perfection. For we have only those moments in time to alleviate the grinding monotony of everyday routine. They light up your life; precious interludes of sweet freedom, wherein the self is reclaimed.

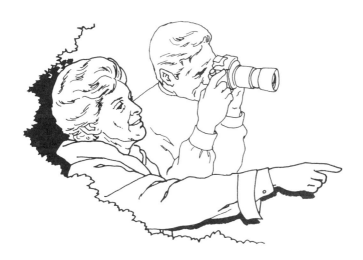

And it needn't be a structured event to make a moment special: the trill of a bird...the fragrance of a flower...the embrace of a friend. Each a nurturing communication to feed your senses and grace your life.

Mirror, mirror on the wall
Who's the fairest one of all?

You, of course. Gamely carrying on in the face of crises and chaos, struggling day by day to keep an untenable situation under control. Performing all the functions of a nurse, cook and therapist with willing hands and most times, a broken heart. Only another caregiver really knows what you are going through. And although caregivers are not looking for compliments or appreciation, I firmly believe they deserve a supportive round of applause, along with a designated CAREGIVERS DAY!

Attitude And Altitude

How high is up? Depends on your attitude: how you organize yourself to face the vicissitudes of each day. Feeling "up" depends on how you visualize the problems: (is the glass half-empty or half full?). Sometimes "up" is measured by small achievements...your relative responds to a new activity, or recognizes people in an old photo, or enjoys a special dessert. Little bits of happiness, but to you they represent something more; tangible evidence of your caring and devotion. How well you have earned that reward! ❧

૨૦

For Men Only

The foregoing strategies and coping techniques
are applicable to both male and female caregivers.
However, there are some situations that require
further briefing for the man who is unaccustomed
to grappling with household care in addition to
assuming the role of caregiver.

Venturing into No Man's Land

You're in strange territory, or so it seems if you've
never had to come face-to-face with a microwave,
vacuum cleaner, washer, dryer and other unusual
appliances.

That was always your partner's domain, but
role-reversal has come full circle and now you're

the man of the house. Don't despair! Help is on the way. Just enlist the services of relatives, friends, and neighbors who will be only too happy to acquaint you with the facts of householding.

"She's All Right"

This form of denial is a normal reaction. Even though you know your spouse is <u>not</u> all right ... that her forgetfulness is becoming more acute, her behavior more unpredictable and sometimes embarrassing to the point where you hesitate to take her anywhere. You may try to cover up for awhile, but soon you'll be forced to admit that the situation is getting out of control. Fortunately, there are viable options right at hand.

Obligation vs. Opportunity

You might feel you're obligating your relatives and friends when you turn to them for help. Keep in mind that helping can offer them an opportunity to ease your burdens, and share in the care of someone they're close to. Don't deny them a chance to show their affection. Your loved one may still sense and enjoy their presence although she is no longer capable of expressing it.

Don't Be Afraid To Ask

Some men have the mistaken perception that asking for assistance implies weakness. Nothing could be further from the truth. Asking for help asserts your masculinity: you're determined to get it right without wasting endless time struggling with problems that could be quickly solved with experienced direction. As the saying goes: seek and ye shall find—the answers. Go for it!

Man Overboard!

The sink or swim syndrome applies...when you feel totally overwhelmed by the complexity of your responsibilities. Just take a deep breath and go with the flow before plunging into an in-depth assessment of your priorities:

- Are you expecting too much of yourself?
- Are you trying to do it all?
- Are you asking for help?
- Are you taking care of your personal needs?
- Are you aware of the available care facilities?

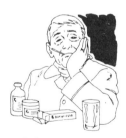

The Life-Saving List

Respite care facilities provide secure professional care while you get a chance to recharge. Whether it's for a day, a weekend or longer period, these facilities offer a safe and constructive environment and allow you some very necessary freedom. Here are the options:

- **Home Care:**
Arrangements with members of the family, friends, visiting nurses or health aides to take care of light meals, housekeeping and laundry while attending to your spouse.

- **Day Care:**
Provides a structured environment along with appropriate activities and entertainment that can prove to be beneficial and stimulating to the patient.

- **Respite Care:**
For a weekend or longer these facilities are professionally staffed for round-the-clock care. Away from the endless caregiving cycle, this respite allows the caregiver time out for a short vacation and a most necessary interval to take care of himself.

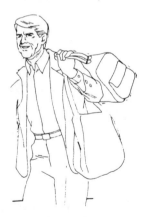

For information regarding these services and Support Groups, call your local Alzheimer's chapter or the National Alzheimer's Association: **1-800-272-3900.**

Are You Putting Your Life On Hold?

Don't! The caregiver who steeps himself in the daily grind without any breaks is heading for a breakdown. No one can endure the relentless stress without suffering mental and physical repercussions. In fairness to yourself and your spouse, arrange time off for your own pleasure.

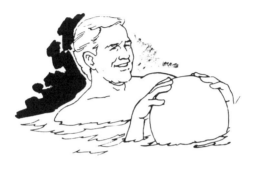

Encourage relationships that stimulate a refreshed perspective as well as enjoyable activities. With male friends, enjoy an evening of cards, bowling, a sports event...an afternoon of golf, tennis, swimming or whatever lifts your spirits and contributes to your peace of mind. With your female friends, relax over a movie or dinner. And hopefully there is a special woman who fills the aching emptiness and satisfies a basic human need for meaningful companionship. Allow these healthy diversions to replenish you mentally and physically. It will improve your performance as a caregiver. And giving dimension to your own life will result in a more effective and loving relationship with your spouse.

To The Man In Her Life

Your spouse, whom you have known and loved most of your life, is sadly on the cusp of cognitive failure. Yet, in all the tragedy of this unforgiving disease, there is a blessing: You!

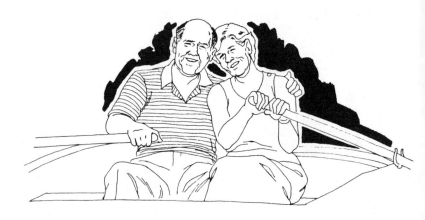

For with your loyalty, steadfastness and commitment, you are helping her through one of life's most devastating trials— even as you suffer the heartbreak of grief and loss. Your devotion is a triumph of the human spirit; a testimonial to the power and glory of love. ❧

છ

SUPPORT GROUPS

In my travels through the torturous maze of Alzheimer's, I found the support group to be my refuge; a place where shared understanding and the calming voice of concerned professionals helped me to continue with renewed courage and spirit. For caregiving is a full-time, back-breaking treadmill of trauma that knows no respite. We're over-burdened and often distraught, silently crying out for some relief. No one is looking for an out...all we want is a chance to get away for a little while to restore tired minds and aching bodies.

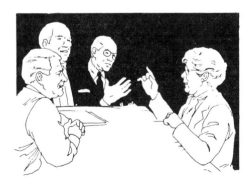

You owe it to the patient to take time out, to have a support network to relieve you. Accepting help is the best thing you can do for your relative since it enables you to stay healthy and continue being of help. Without this assistance, you will collapse under the strain.

And so the support group becomes our rich sustaining ally, offering safe haven where we can ventilate pent-up feelings, release tensions and gain a more objective focus on our stress. This sensitive, reassuring guidance brightens perspective and lifts morale. Counselors offer invaluable assistance with their knowledge of social services, Medicare and Medicaid programs, and other agencies designed to make life easier.

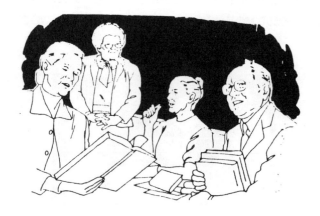

Shared communication of daily experiences teaches us how to cope more effectively with our patients. Just as important, we are reminded to care for ourselves with regular checkups, mammograms and other procedures. I find it tragic that many caregivers reject the tremendous advantages of this network because of a reluctance to expose the frailties of a dear one to "outsiders" — as though it were an act of betrayal. There are no "outsiders" here; only the embattled corps of caregivers united in a common cause: the ceaseless fight against a ravaging disease.

My own participation in a support group was at the Wien Center for Alzheimer's Disease at Mt. Sinai Medical Center, Miami Beach. Our relatives received evaluation and diagnosis while we were given counseling, nurturing and educational advice that were indispensable.

It was a heartwarming, enriching experience with all of us becoming an extended family. We became very comfortable together. We even learned to laugh and inject a little humor into some of the situations we faced. Through the years many of us remained close friends, meeting for weekly lunches, keeping in touch with mutual concerns. And when tragedy struck with the loss of a loved one, our caregiver friends were there for us. Somehow, the bond that was forged through hardship and sorrow became a symbol of strength and solace.

Some Facts About Support Groups

- Support groups are free of charge.

- There are groups for caregivers in all states. Call your local Alzheimer's Association and they will refer you to one in your area. If a support group isn't available, consider starting one yourself.

- Support groups usually consist of any where from six to twelve members.

- Meetings are usually held monthly or bimonthly.

- Many support groups provide information about community resources which you might not otherwise learn about.

- Support groups are also available for people in the early stages of Alzheimer's. Your local association will know if there is a suitable one for your relative. ✒

ɞ

THE WAY YOU WERE
AND CAN BE AGAIN!

You may have completely forsaken the creative talents and absorbing interests that once were so much a part of your life. But they are not hopelessly lost, just neglected. You owe it to yourself to make time for the pursuit of pleasure.

For you are a dimensional person, with a vital essence of your being crying out for personal expression, for activities that make life more meaningful. So whatever it is, do your thing! You will achieve self-fulfillment with the adrenalizing energy that comes from your accomplishments. Just to prod you into action, here are a few reminders of the way you were, and can be again:

Creative Cook

Visions of sugarplums, chocolate mousse, and the exotic variety of your own secret concoctions that filled the house with tantalizing aromas. And how about those yummy casseroles that turned leftovers into culinary triumphs (good enough for company!). You were queen of the kitchen, no small accomplishment when you remember how everyone looked forward to your dinners, and tried

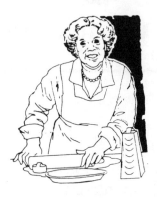

to coax the mysteries of your recipes from your secret file. Yes, those were the days. Bring 'em back alive!

Designing Lady

Are you the gal who used to sew her own smashing originals...and wouldn't you enjoy hearing those compliments again? All it takes is a little persuasive needling to get you right back on track.

For talent like yours shouldn't be wasted, and there's not a moment to lose. Get out that sewing box and make your designer-dreams come true. With lustrous satins and vibrant silks whipped into stunning fashions under the magic of your artistic fingers. Those enthusiastic compliments are on the way!

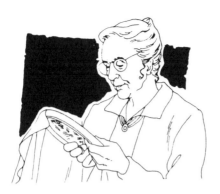

Knit-To-Fit

Remember the soothing click-click of those busy needles as you knit 'n purled something spectacular...and what a calming influence it was.

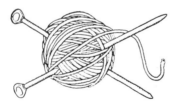

And how everyone admired your beautiful wardrobe of plush sweaters and magnificent dresses. And let's not forget the warm and wonderful little socks and booties you donated to the Children's Hospital for needy babies. Happily, knitting is a delightfully portable hobby; you can take it with you.

Green Thumber

Lucky you, with all those radiant flowers and lusty plants...and a houseful of nature's beauty to prove it! But you were always gifting friends with the bounty of your efforts.

And you didn't let it go at that: you matched each plant with an attractively decorated ceramic pot which you hand-painted yourself. How long has it been since you made time for this lovely, absorbing interest that gave you so much pleasure. Certainly you must miss it. But don't just miss it, do it!

Sports Scene

Is it golf, swimming, aerobics, walking? Take your pick and enjoy the exhilaration of tone-up and pare-down exercises.

A refreshing walk in the open air, a few laps around the pool, a half-hour with aerobics on TV...all calculated to reduce stress and release emotional build-up. And whether it's a stationary bike, slant board, treadmaster or any other vehicle, exercise invigorates and does wonders for your mental attitude.

Play It Again, Pam:

Dust off the piano, haul out the guitar, the violin or whatever your favorite instrument happens to be and bring back the old feeling.

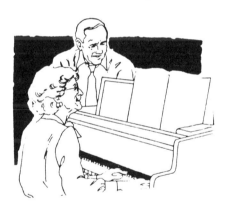

Nothing is more relaxing than music, especially when you are the artist. Maybe you haven't thought about it lately, but think about it now...how calming, how soul-satisfying it was to just sit down and play. And how it seemed to re-energize your mind and body. The delight of playing again can be enhanced with a few lessons to reinforce your confidence and restore your musical self.

The Right Time To Write

It's now. Think of how you used to fill in your diary, write letters, sketch out a story line to be finished later— the 'later' that never came. There's no time like the present to get back into the habit of doing something creative and mentally challenging. And it's not a question of how much time: it's what you do with the time you have.

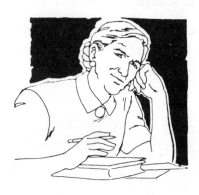

Adapting yourself to the discipline of writing will take determination and persistence. But how worthwhile it is!

Read 'N Relax

If you loved to read, you were always up on all the current best sellers, positive-thinking magazines and how-to manuals. Sadly you've let it all go. You need this stimulation now more than ever to lift your spirit, strengthen morale, and give you fresh perspective. New trends and provocative ideas stir the imagination and help you to withstand the difficult routine that caregiving exacts.

Dance Your Troubles Away

Maybe you think you've forgotten how to put one foot in front of the other — that time has put lead in your feet, and stilled the song in your heart. Just think again and head for the nearest dance class. There are so many available, just waiting for you to brush-up and start tripping the light fantastic like you used to. A little practice, and voila! You're turning and twirling gracefully as ever, and having a wonderful time. Need we say more!

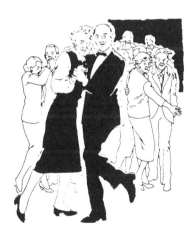

This section has outlined only a few suggestions for renewal. Add your own ideas and get moving with your projects. Rediscover a fount of well-deserved personal enrichment and satisfaction. The immediate goal: to make some time each day dedicated to yourself. &

REACHING OUT

ð

THE NURSING HOME DECISION

Although you're frantically doing the best you can, you realize you're losing ground. Your relative is becoming unmanageable and there are times when you feel you can't go on. Yet with almost superhuman determination, you continue, becoming hopelessly lost in a maelstrom of indecisions. You're afraid to give up; afraid to face the future; afraid to admit what is happening. To save the patient and yourself, you must recognize the need for immediate help.

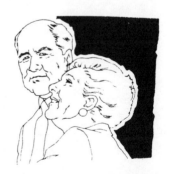

As your loved one's condition becomes more and more unmanageable, the threatening shadow of the nursing home becomes a reality. If you have not already done so, check out the local day care centers, respite facilities, in-home health care workers, aides and nursing homes. Anguish and despair are common emotions at this time. Your concern, your caring is shown every day in so many ways. But as agitation, loss of control, and other disabilities develop, you experience the ambivalence of a perfectly human love-hate response — along with a sense of disloyalty and dooming failure. All destructive, misplaced emotions.

For you have done everything you could. Now you must recognize the crisis for what it is: the illness has progressed far beyond your capabilities and decisions must be made. A structured environment will permit your loved one to save her dignity. It will allow you to save your sanity.

Knowing When To Stop

The hardest decision to reach is knowing when you're in a no-win situation, with you and your relative at an impasse. Problems have escalated into refusal to eat, to bathe, to do anything that requires a certain amount of patient-participation.

Aggressive behavior and physical infirmities demand immediate professional assistance. You have come as far as you can with vigilance and courage. There can be no turning back, for the sake of your loved one, and for your own sanity.

These signs indicate when it is time to seek a nursing home:

- The patient refuses food, throwing it on the floor.

- He/she will not bathe and fights off any efforts at coaxing.

- Medication is flatly refused on a continual basis.

- The patient's aggressive behavior pattern intensifies.

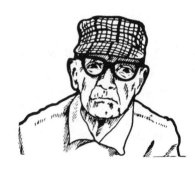

Pride And Prejudice

I have heard caregivers announce proudly, "I would never send my mother to a nursing home!" But never is a long, long time and the day may come when refusing to consider other options becomes a disservice to the patient. Not to mention protracted and futile bondage for the caregiver. When a patient's deterioration mandates custodial care and almost constant attention, a nursing home may be the only solution. And not just any nursing home.

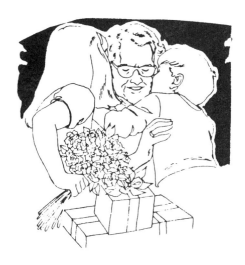

Criticism of nursing homes abounds these days—much of it justified. However there are many well-managed, competently administered homes and hopefully you will be able to locate one in your area. Tough love comes into its own, even where Alzheimer's patients are concerned. And that's because we love them enough to let them go.

The Conflict Of Interest

The caregiver of a growing family brought her impaired parent home to stay with them. At the outset this seemed like a feasible and convenient arrangement. But soon, discord began to surface. The teenagers resented curtailing their home-activities and hated having to share a room. The husband, usually affable and cooperative, was disturbed at the restrictions. He felt neglected and that his wife no longer seemed to have time for him.

In a situation like this, the caregiver suffers most, torn between her love and devotion for her family and her ill parent. This powerful conflict of emotions simply adds to her confusion and burden of responsibilities. And it's not that the family has suddenly become insensitive and callous. They are reacting to the disruptions and displacements that have changed their lives.

Consultations with a therapist helps present an objective perspective that might alleviate some of the family's concerns and tensions. But as the patient's condition worsens, the caregiver endures the almost intolerable mental strain of knowing that a decision must be made. Sadly, there are few choices, but when the fractious environment threatens to destroy the household, a realistic solution must be found. That is the caregiver's hardest task of all. But just as she has met all the other challenges with courage and faith, those strong convictions will see her through this, too.

How To Select A Nursing Home

When it's time to select a nursing home, investigate! Become an informed caregiver for your own peace of mind and the well-being of your relative. These guidelines will help you to select a nursing home.

• Visit the nursing home at mealtimes, (arrange to eat a meal there) and ask about activities and regularly scheduled programs.

- Observe the attitude of staff members.
- Question supervisors, nurses aides and physicians.
- Talk to other caregivers about how they find the quality of care in the facility.
- Ask yourself these questions:
  - Are the bedrooms and communal areas clean and cheerful?
  - Is the professional staff well-qualified and communicative?
  - Are the service people and aides patient and helpful?
  - Are the meals nutritious and nicely served?
  - Is the facility currently state-licensed?
  - Are fire exits and stairs conveniently accessible?
  - Is management reputable and financially stable?

**For further information
you can call the toll-free
Elder Helpline (800) 262-2243** ⁊

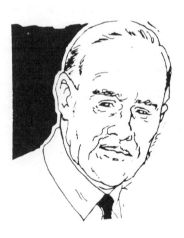

AFTER THE NURSING HOME

There is no easy transition from home to the nursing home. And you, the anguished caregiver, suffer more than your patient. Feeling you have abandoned your loved one to the care of strangers, you suffer excruciating pangs of guilt and remorse. Even though professional assistance was necessary, you perceive this step as a personal failure.

The fact that there was no alternative is now obscured under suffocating layers of the "if only's"— "if only I had waited"... "if only I'd been more patient." The "if only" syndrome is always destructive, demoralizing and futile, since in your heart you know you could no longer cope with the situation. Yet you continue to live in a state of mourning that seems to have no relief, no solace. But there is relief to alleviate your emotional gridlock. As always, your support group stands ready to guide you through this traumatic period. Allow yourself the compassionate understanding of those who have endured the same torment, and who know what it is to let go — and then go on with their lives.

The comfort of friends and relatives helps ease your pain, even if it's only a shoulder to cry on, or a reminiscence to share. The caregiver who isolates herself is heading for depression and other serious health problems. Learn to be gentle with yourself, remembering that you did all you possibly could until it was no longer possible. And remember too, that separation does not mean alienation. You are free to visit, able to do what you can to make your loved one's life brighter and more livable.

The reassuring familiarity of your presence is important to your relative. And in time, the healing will take place with warm and wonderful recollections that become a legacy of love.

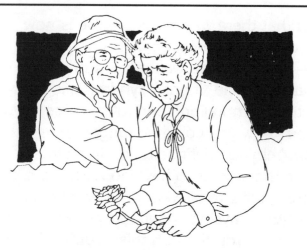

Ideas For Visiting With The Patient

- Keep visits short and cheerful so as not to overtire the patient.

- Bring little treats to enliven the day.

- Read short passages from an uplifting book.

- Go for a walk; if your relative is not ambulatory take her outside in the wheelchair for a change of scene.

- Listen sympathetically to complaints, keeping in mind that facts and fantasies are often confused. If you sense there is a valid reason for a complaint, investigate!

- Expect good days and bad days and learn to bridge the difference with courage and faith.☙

è&

THE LAST WORD

I sincerely hope this little book has helped you
realize the extent of your capabilities, and to
respect the boundaries of your limitations. As
every caregiver knows, caregiving is a way of life.
But it must be handled with some objectivity to
achieve a healthy balance. Otherwise, by allowing
the sum total of your duties to dominate your
every moment, you risk becoming a casualty too.

I recommend that you keep this book handy to
guide you through the dark days. And let me
remind you once again that there are people
and places to turn to: Alzheimer's Associations;
support groups; day care centers; in-home health
care workers; Medicare and Medicaid assistance
plans; respite facilities; aides, and when indicated,
the nursing home.

To you, to all the Captains courageous who are
waging a daily battle against the havoc and heartbreak of Alzheimer's, I send my fervent hopes and
prayers with the pain of deep understanding and
heartfelt compassion. è&

CAREGIVERS PRAYER

Dear God, help me through another day
to face problems known and unknown
Grant me sensitivity and understanding
so that I can cope gently with
my loved one, who rails at life with
bitter accusations and assails me
with recriminations that I know have
no basis in reality.

The harsh words are not really meant
for me – the bewildering actions
are totally the disordered trauma of
this cruelty; this devastating
disease that has trapped my loved one
in its merciless grip.

How well I know – but sometimes knowledge
fails me and I become frustrated,
impatient and unkind – for Lord, I'm
one of your imperfect children, too
with a broken heart, a tired body and
an oppressed mind – but
I'll go on and on believing, as I
hope and pray that somehow,
somewhere, there will be a cure
one day.

Florian Raymond ❧

APPENDIX 1
IMPORTANT ADDRESSES

Alzheimer's Association,
919 N Michigan Ave., Suite 1000,
Chicago, IL. 60611-1676.
Phone toll-free: 1-800-272-3900.

*The Alzheimer's Association has listings of
over 1,200 support groups and 190 chapters
nationwide, providing support and assistance
to patients and their families.*

Alzheimer's Disease Society of Canada,
491 Lawrence Ave West, #501,
Toronto, Ontario, Canada M5M 1C7.

Alzheimer's Disease Education and Referral Center,
PO Box 8250, Silver Springs, MD. 20907-8250.
301-495-3311 ॐ

APPENDIX 2
USEFUL BOOKS

Grandpa Doesn't Know It's Me
by Donna W Guthrie.
Publisher: Human Sciences Press Inc.,
233 Spring St., New York, N.Y. 10013
Recommended for pre-school through fifth grade.

Sachiko Means Happiness
by Kimiko Sakai.
Publisher: Childrens Book Press
1461 9th Ave., San Francisco, CA. 94422
Recommended for kindergarten through fifth grade.

The 36-Hour Day
by Nancy L. Mace and Peter V. Rabins.
Publisher: Johns Hopkins University Press
Baltimore and London.
A practical family guide for the care of persons with Alzheimer's and related disorders. ક્ષ

ª

Appendix 3
The Caregivers Series

**Failure-Free Activities
for the Alzheimer's Patient**
by Carmel Sheridan

This award-winning book shows you how to raise
the quality of life for patient and caregiver through
simple, meaningful activities. The author describes
how to focus on the abilities that remain rather
than the person's deficits. Hundreds of activities
are outlined which help to raise self-esteem and
relieve boredom and frustration
$10.95

**Reminiscence: Uncovering
A Lifetime of Memories**
by Carmel Sheridan

Written in easily-understood language, this book
shows how to use reminiscence with the well and
the confused elderly in the home, in day care, in
social centers and hospitals. 164 pages packed
with activities and ways to uncover memories.
$11.95

Living In The Labyrinth: A Personal Journey Through The Maze of Alzheimer's Disease
by Diana Friel McGowin

Written by a relatively young woman who was diagnosed with early-onset Alzheimer's, this book describes the coping mechanisms she developed for plain survival. Living In The Labyrinth gives unique insight into the inner world and feelings of the person with Alzheimer's disease.
$10.95

The Alzheimer's Family Manual
by Lyle Weinstein

An essential audio cassette program for family and friends of patients and caregivers. Set out in simple terms, the manual shows how to approach the painful effects of the disease with sanity, kindness and simplicity.
$11.95

The Caregivers Catalog

This free catalog is full of information on helpful books and activity resources dealing with Alzheimer's disease. Many of the activity resources, including video and musical tapes, help to stimulate reminiscence and memory-sharing.

If you would like a free copy of the Caregiver's Catalog, please complete and mail the form on the following page. ❧

ॐ

ORDER FORM

Mail To:
Elder Books
PO Box 490, Forest Knolls, CA. 94933

Quantity	Title	Price
_____	Surviving Alzheimer's A Guide for Families	$10.95
_____	Failure Free Activities for the Alzheimer's Patient	$10.95
_____	Reminiscence	$11.95
_____	The Alzheimer's Family Manual	$11.95
_____	Living In The Labyrinth: A Journey Through The Maze of Alzheimer's	$10.95
_____	The Caregivers Catalog	**FREE**

Name: _____

Address:_____

City:_____

State_____ Zip:_____

Shipping: $2.50 for first book.
Additional books: $.75 each.
California residents please add 8.5% California Sales Tax ॐ